I0696374

Contents

Understanding the Carnivore Diet 7

What is the Carnivore Diet? 7

Origins and Evolution of the Carnivore Diet 7

Benefits and Controversies of the Carnivore Diet

....8

How the Carnivore Diet Works......................10

Getting Started with the Carnivore Diet 12

Preparing Yourself Mentally and Emotionally ...12

Assessing Your Health and Goals 12

Transitioning to the Carnivore Diet................13

Common Challenges and How to Overcome Them

....14

What Is The Carnivore Diet: Health Myths, Side

Effects And Pseudoscience 16

1. What is a carnivore diet? 18

2. The carnivore diet plan: fuel vs macronutrients

.... 20

Dietary fiber: a carnivore diet myth 22

Carbs: flawed carnivore diet reasoning 23

The Difference Between Carbs And Sugar 24

3. Carnivore diet menu 26

Carnivore diet food list 27

4. Carnivore diet benefits 28

Carnivore diet weight loss 28

5. Carnivore diet side effects 29

Parchment Baked Lemon Salmon & Vegetables

Recipe...30

Chicken and Zucchini Noodle Salad Recipe......34

Fish Tacos Recipe. 37

Cauliflower Curry Recipe. 43

Curried Chicken Bowl Recipe.........................47

Mashed Cauliflower with Rosemary Recipe......51

Braised Brussels Sprouts Recipe. 53

Coconut Bread Stuffing Recipe. 55

Roast Turkey with Sage Pesto Recipe. 58

Moroccan Stir Fry Recipe. 62

Celeriac Soup Recipe. 66

Tarragon Chicken and Leeks Recipe. 69

Tasty Salmon Bowl With Arugula Dressing Recipe.

....73

Asian Steak Kebabs Recipe. 78

Kimchi Meatballs Recipe. 82

Buckwheat And Brussels Sprout Salad Recipe. 86

Satay Chicken Bowl With Almond Sauce Recipe.

....90

Thai Quinoa Recipe. 96

Yellow Squash Noodles with Meatballs and Olive

Tapenade Recipe. 100

Sardine Nicoise Salad Recipe. 106

Oven Roasted Artichokes with Lemon and Olive

Oil Dipping Sauce Recipe....................110

Cool Sardine Salad Recipe. 113

Ajvar Dip Recipe....................117

Buckwheat Ravioli Recipe. 119

Nachos With Rutabaga Chips Recipe. 125

Understanding the Carnivore Diet

What is the Carnivore Diet?

The Carnivore Diet is a dietary approach that emphasizes the consumption of animal-based foods while excluding most or all plant-based foods. It is a highly restrictive diet that primarily consists of meat, fish, eggs, and animal fats. The concept behind the Carnivore Diet is rooted in the belief that our ancestors predominantly consumed animal foods and that humans are biologically adapted to thrive on a meat-based diet.

Origins and Evolution of the Carnivore Diet

The idea of consuming an exclusively animal-based diet has been present in various cultures throughout history. However, the modern resurgence of the Carnivore Diet can be attributed to the work of Dr. Shawn Baker, a prominent advocate and proponent of the diet. Dr. Baker, along with other proponents, argues that the Carnivore Diet can help improve health, promote weight loss, and address certain health conditions.

Benefits and Controversies of the Carnivore Diet

Supporters of the Carnivore Diet claim numerous benefits, including weight loss, improved mental clarity, increased energy levels, reduced inflammation, and better digestion. They argue that the elimination of carbohydrates and plant-based foods can alleviate certain health conditions such as autoimmune disorders, digestive issues, and metabolic disorders. Additionally, proponents highlight the simplicity of the diet and the potential for decreased food cravings and improved satiety.

However, the Carnivore Diet is not without its controversies. Critics argue that the diet lacks essential nutrients and may lead to nutritional deficiencies, particularly in vitamins, minerals, and fiber that are commonly found in plant-based foods. They express concerns about the long-term health implications, such as an increased risk of heart disease, due to the high intake of saturated fats and cholesterol. Additionally, the diet's environmental impact and ethical considerations related to animal welfare are subjects of debate.

How the Carnivore Diet Works

The Carnivore Diet operates on the principle that by eliminating plant-based foods and relying solely on animal-based foods, the body can enter a state of nutritional ketosis. Nutritional ketosis occurs when the body transitions from using glucose as its primary fuel source to utilizing ketones derived from fat metabolism. By restricting carbohydrates and reducing insulin levels, the body is prompted to burn stored fat for energy, leading to potential weight loss.

Getting Started with the Carnivore Diet

Preparing Yourself Mentally and Emotionally

Before embarking on the Carnivore Diet, it is important to mentally and emotionally prepare yourself for the significant dietary changes. Understand the reasons behind your decision and set realistic expectations. Educate yourself about the diet, its potential benefits, and challenges to ensure you are fully informed and committed.

Assessing Your Health and Goals

Evaluate your current health status and consult with a healthcare professional or a registered dietitian to assess whether the Carnivore Diet is suitable for you. Consider your health goals and objectives, such as weight loss, improved energy levels, or addressing specific health conditions. It is essential to have a clear understanding of what you hope to achieve through this dietary approach.

Transitioning to the Carnivore Diet

Transitioning to the Carnivore Diet should be done gradually to allow your body to adjust to the new way of eating. Start by eliminating processed foods, sugars, grains, and legumes from your diet. Gradually reduce the consumption of fruits, vegetables, and other plant-based foods while increasing your intake of animal-based foods. This gradual transition can help minimize potential digestive discomfort and withdrawal symptoms.

Common Challenges and How to Overcome Them

The Carnivore Diet may present certain challenges, especially during the initial adaptation period. Some individuals may experience cravings for eliminated foods or encounter difficulties in social situations where plant-based options are prevalent. To overcome these challenges, it is crucial to plan and prepare your meals in advance, find suitable substitutes for favorite foods, and communicate your dietary needs with friends and family. Seek support from online communities or connect with individuals who follow a similar dietary approach for guidance and encouragement.

Understanding the Carnivore Diet is the foundation for successfully implementing this dietary approach. By familiarizing yourself with its principles, origins, benefits, and controversies, you can make informed decisions regarding your health and well-being. Remember to consult with a healthcare professional before making any significant dietary changes and tailor the diet to suit your individual needs and goals.

What Is The Carnivore Diet: Health Myths, Side Effects And Pseudoscience

Is your life not hard enough? Would you like to deplete your body's reserves and deprive it of essential nutrients to lose a few pounds? Meet the carnivore diet, a fad that's bad for your health, your wallet and your self-esteem.

The carnivore diet is the shiniest fad diet on the block. It's not new, it's not even original, but it is Bear Grylls extreme (though we doubt Bear Grylls would ever endorse this diet). But if you're into magic beans and conspiracy theories, it might just be the perfect diet for you.

Sadly, your body won't agree because this diet completely overlooks the body's essential nutrition needs. It parades pseudoscience as fact, promising that a meat-only diet will cure everything from autism to alcoholism.

To be clear, there is no carnivore diet science. Instead, this fad presents non-specific medical research as proof to convince people that it's the magic bullet for a six-pack and eternal life. In this article, we review the carnivore diet claims and explain exactly why you should stay away from it.

☝ DISCLAIMER ☝

This article is for informational purposes only. It is not intended to constitute or be a substitute for professional medical advice, diagnosis, or treatment.

1. What is a carnivore diet?

The carnivore diet is a zero-carb diet that spreads misinformation about antinutrients in plant foods — a belief shared by many fad diets including the paleo diet and the blood type diet. Lectins, they claim, are evil antinutrients in plants that make people fat.

Say goodbye to fruit, vegetables, grains, starches, nuts, and legumes because the carnivore diet dictates that you can only eat meat, animal fat, and eggs.

Rather than targeting proven causes of obesity,

weight gain, and diabetes, like refined sugars and fast food, carnivore diet gurus incorrectly accuse lectins — proteins found in raw beans, lentils and grains. But lectins are eliminated by baking and boiling, which makes them perfectly safe to eat.

However, there's plenty of evidence to suggest that we are not eating enough of these fiber-rich plant foods. Lectins are not a problem. If they were, obesity and diabetes would be very old health problems, but they're not. These are diseases of our century.

2. The carnivore diet plan: fuel vs macronutrients

The carnivore diet is a more extreme version of the keto diet. The goal is to cut out glucose and turbocharge the body's fat-burning capabilities to replace the lost fuel and make up for the lack of glucose — a process called ketogenesis.

The body stores excess carbs as fat. When blood sugar levels drop, it starts to break down fat stores, and cells can then turn fatty acids into ketones — an alternative source of energy for most cells (except the liver and red blood cells).

However, this theory conveniently forgets that your body doesn't just need energy — it needs other stuff too. Every chemical reaction is regulated by a range of nutrients, including sodium, potassium, calcium, vitamins, and antioxidants. We get most of these from our diet.

So when you cut out food groups, you're restricting your micronutrient intake too. Let's take the vegan diet as an example: nutrient deficiencies aren't caused by eating too many vegetables, they're caused by cutting out whole food groups. The same logic applies to the carnivore diet.

Dietary fiber: a carnivore diet myth

Proponents advocate with cult-like fanaticism that your body doesn't need fiber. This is totally incorrect. Fiber is a critical part of a healthy diet, and there's plenty of science to prove it.

Here are some important dietary fiber benefits:

- preventing constipation — a common problem in keto-based diets.

- removing excess cholesterols and bile acids from your body

- regulating blood glucose and blood lipid levels

- supporting immune system health

- feeding the essential bacteria in your gut microbiome

This last point is not to be underestimated — scientists even call this ecosystem of microorganisms a 'new organ'. Good bacteria in your gut help prevent infections, and they produce vital nutrients (like butyrate) that fuel the cells of your gut lining.

A happy and balanced gut microbiome even helps regulate body weight, but these microbes thrive on prebiotics — dietary fibers and nutrients found in plants — which are often completely absent from the carnivore diet.

Carbs: flawed carnivore diet reasoning

Carbs are the devil in this diet, a position that

defies common sense: your body depends on carbs for energy. Your brain is mainly fueled by glucose and carbs give your muscles energy, so when you go cold turkey, your brain doesn't work as well, neither do your muscles because they are hungry.

The Difference Between Carbs And Sugar

Unfortunately, carbs are very unpopular nowadays because they have been linked to serious deadly diseases: obesity, diabetes, and heart disease. But not all carbs are bad! Refined carbs in fast food, sugary beverages, and chocolate bars are nothing like the carbs in whole grains, beans, fruit and veg.

Whole, unprocessed carbohydrates are good for your body. They are packed with nutrients, fibers, and resistant starches that make you feel fuller for longer. Complex carbs keep your blood sugar levels stable, while providing nutrition for your cells and your gut bacteria.

The carnivore diet would have you believe that all carbs are evil and your carb cravings must be eliminated. That's simply not true. Your body would benefit more from a balanced diet with whole grains, beans, fruit and vegetables, than bingeing on meat, bacon and eggs.

As microbiome expert Miguel Torribio-Mateas

points out: "Scientists have found that when an Inuit swaps carnivore meals for a typical American diet (like tacos or fried chicken with fries), their microbiome becomes Western very rapidly, and their risk of becoming obese and diabetic increases too."

3. Carnivore diet menu

Now, let's take a look at the list of foods on the carnivore diet and think about how this will affect your digestion and your monthly budget. Carnivore diet gurus recommend that you only choose the highest quality of meat, such as grass-fed beef, and wild line-caught salmon.

Carnivore diet food list

- red meat

- white meat

- offal (i.e., organ meat)

- animal fat (i.e., lard)

- poultry

- fish

- seafood

- eggs

- dairy (optional)

Like other restrictive fads, a zero-carb diet will likely fuel cravings for other foods (probably junk food). This increases the risk of bingeing, unnecessary shame, and abandoning your goal of getting healthier. Plus, restrictive diets are associated with eating disorder tendencies.

4. Carnivore diet benefits

There is a treasure trove of seemingly magical weight loss carnivore diet before and after transformations online. The same websites claim that people have recovered from every kind of imaginable disease too. And yet, there's no evidence to suggest that the carnivore diet has any health benefits whatsoever.

Carnivore diet weight loss

There are no proven carnivore diet benefits

Yes, you can lose weight on the carnivore diet because it is an extreme diet that deprives you of adequate nutrition. However, extreme weight loss also comes with a yoyo effect. Sure, you lose the weight, but many people end up putting it back on and getting even heavier.

5. Carnivore diet side effects

There are short-term and long-term carnivore diet side effects. At first, you may experience a set of symptoms known as the keto flu that are caused by depriving your body of glucose.

Short-term side effects

Nausea Vomiting

Headache Fluid imbalances

Fatigue Dizziness

Insomnia Constipation

Short-term symptoms last a few days to a few weeks and are unpleasant. They can result in fluid and electrolyte imbalances. These are serious because they are a sign that your body lacks essential micronutrients that allow your cells to function normally.

Parchment Baked Lemon Salmon & Vegetables Recipe.

Ingredients

* 1 small zucchini, julienne sliced

* 1 scallion, julienne sliced

* 1 boneless, skinless salmon fillet, about 4 ounces

* Salt and pepper

* 1 tsp. lemon zest, divided

* 2 tsp. extra-virgin olive oil, divided

* Fresh lemon slices

* Fresh dill

Instructions

1. Preheat oven to 400 degrees.

2. Take a piece of parchment paper, about 12 x 15 inches, and fold the long side in half. Form a crease, then open out flat. [SEP]

3. Arrange julienne sliced zucchini and green onion in the middle on one side of the crease. Sprinkle vegetables with a bit of salt and pepper, and half of the lemon zest, then drizzle all over with half of the olive oil. [SEP]

4. Lay salmon fillet on top of vegetables. Season it with salt, pepper, and the remaining lemon zest and olive oil. [SEP]

5. Now fold the parchment over to cover ingredients. Starting at the bottom folded corner, begin folding the edges of the parchment together,

making small overlapping folds every 1 to 2 inches. Continue folding all the way around to create a half moon shaped package. Fold the ends again to make sure they are sealed.

6. Place parchment package on a baking sheet and bake until package has puffed, about 12 to 15 minutes. Transfer package to a plate, open and serve immediately. Garnish with fresh lemon slices and fresh dill.

Chicken and Zucchini Noodle Salad Recipe.

Ingredients

* 1 chicken breast half, boneless and skinless

* Juice of a lemon, divided

* Salt, pepper

* 1 tsp. dried oregano

* 1 Tbsp. olive oil

* 1 medium zucchini, cut into noodles

* 1/2 cup cherry tomatoes, halved

* 2 Tbsp. pine nuts

* 2 Tbsp. minced fresh basil

Instructions

1. Place chicken breast half between 2 sheets of waxed paper and pound to a 1/2 inch thickness. Sprinkle both sides with half the lemon juice, then season both sides with salt, pepper and dried oregano.

2. In a medium size skillet, heat oil over medium high heat. Sauté chicken breast half for 3 to 4 minutes per side or until juices run clear. Remove from pan to a warm plate.

3. Cut zucchini into noodles using a spiralizer,

julienne peeler or mandoline, then place noodles in a large bowl. [SEP]

4. Add cherry tomato halves, pine nuts and minced basil to bowl, then toss to combine. [SEP]

5. Slice chicken breast half into 3/4 inch thick strips. Add chicken strips to bowl, sprinkle with remaining lemon juice and season with salt and pepper to taste. [SEP]

6. Toss the salad one more time to combine all ingredients, then serve

Fish Tacos Recipe.

Ingredients

Fish Fillets

* 3 Tbsp. oil, such as olive or coconut, melted

* 1/2 lb. fish fillets

* 2 Tbsp. coconut flour

* 2 Tbsp. arrowroot powder

* A good pinch each of salt, pepper, and paprika

Tortillas

* 1/4 cup coconut flour

* 1 cup arrowroot powder

* 1 Tbsp. golden flaxseed meal

* 1/4 tsp. salt

* 1 1/4 cup unsweetened coconut, almond or flaxseed milk

* 2 eggs

* Oil, such as olive or coconut, for frying

* Shredded cabbage, green and purple

* Diced avocado cubes

* Thinly sliced scallions

* Finely minced cilantro

* Lime wedges

Lime Crema

* 1 cup plain yogurt or kefir

* Fresh lime juice (1/4/ lime)

* A good pinch each of salt, cumin, and paprika

Instructions

Directions for fish fillets

1. Preheat oven to 400 degrees F (205 degrees C). Drizzle a rimmed baking sheet with 1 tablespoon oil, set aside.

2. On a shallow plate, combine coconut flour, arrowroot powder, salt, pepper and paprika, stir with a fork to combine.

3. Coat fish fillets with flour mixture, transfer to baking sheet and drizzle fillets with remaining 2 tablespoons of oil.

4. Bake fish fillets until cooked through, about 20 minutes, flipping halfway through baking.

Remove fillets from oven and set aside.

Directions for tortillas

1. In a medium bowl add coconut flour, arrowroot powder, golden flaxseed meal and salt, whisk to combine.

2. Make a well in the center of the flour mixture. Add milk and eggs and whisk batter until thoroughly combined.

3. Let tortilla batter rest for a few minutes, as coconut flour absorbs moisture and thickens slightly.

4. Heat about a half teaspoon of oil in a skillet over medium heat. Pour 1/4 cup of tortilla batter

into the center of the skillet. With an off set spatula or the back of a spoon, smooth out batter to create an 6 inch tortilla.

5. Fry tortilla for about 2 minutes on each side. Repeat process with remaining batter, adding another half teaspoon of oil to the skillet for each tortilla. This makes about 8 tortillas.

6. To assemble tacos, first top each tortilla with shredded cabbage. Then cut the fish fillets into bite size pieces and divide equally among the tacos.

7. Garnish each taco with cubed avocado, sliced scallions, and finely minced cilantro. Finish off with a drizzle of Lime Crema (see below) and a

squeeze of fresh lime juice.

Directions for lime crema

1. Combine all ingredients in a small bowl, whisk
to combine.

Cauliflower Curry Recipe.

Ingredients

* 2 Tbsp. oil, such as coconut or olive

* 1/4 cup diced onion

* 2 stalks celery, thinly sliced

* 1 clove garlic, minced

* 1/2 tsp. powdered coriander

* 1/2 tsp. powdered cumin

* 1/2 tsp. powdered ginger

* 1/2 tsp. powdered turmeric

* 1/4 tsp. red pepper flakes

* 1 cauliflower, about 1 1/2 pounds, cut into bite

size pieces

* 1 zucchini, halved lengthwise, then sliced into

half moons about 1/2 inch thick

* 3 tomatoes, diced

* 1 tsp. salt

* 2 cups water or vegetable broth

* 2 handfuls baby spinach leaves

* 2 Tbsp. toasted slivered almonds

* 2 Tbsp. fresh cilantro, finely minced

* 1 lemon cut into wedges

* Plain yogurt (optional)

Instructions

1. In a cooking pot or large skillet, heat oil over medium heat.

2. Add diced onions and sliced celery, saute about 5 minutes.

3. Now add minced garlic and continue to saute

vegetables for another 5 minutes or until vegetables are softened.

4. Next add the powdered spices, coriander, cumin, ginger, turmeric and the red pepper flakes, stir to combine and saute until spices are fragrant, about 1 minute.

5. Now add the cauliflower pieces, zucchini half moons, diced tomatoes, salt and water or broth.

6. Bring to a boil over high heat, then reduce heat to medium low, cover and simmer until cauliflower is tender, about 20 minutes.

7. Uncover, add spinach and simmer for another 3 to 4 minutes. Season to taste with additional salt and pepper if needed.

8. Garnish curry with a sprinkling of toasted slivered almonds and finely minced cilantro. Serve with lemon wedges and a few dollops of plain yogurt (optional).

Curried Chicken Bowl Recipe.

Ingredients

* 2 tablespoons olive oil

* 2 tablespoons canned coconut milk

* 1 tablespoon fresh lemon juice

* 1/2 teaspoon minced garlic

* 1/2 teaspoon powdered turmeric

* 1/2 teaspoon powdered ginger

* 1/4 teaspoon powdered stevia

* Salt and pepper to taste

Salad

* 1 1/2 cups cooked chicken, white or dark meat, shredded or cubed

* 1/4 cup diced celery

* 1/4 cup diced Granny Smith apple

* 2 tablespoons finely chopped red onion

* 2 tablespoons slivered almonds

* 1 cup fresh spinach leaves

* 1 cup cooked quinoa

* Fresh cilantro for garnish

Instructions

1. To make dressing, in a small bowl add olive oil, canned coconut milk, fresh lemon juice, minced garlic, powdered turmeric, powdered ginger, powdered stevia, salt and pepper. Whisk to

combine, set dressing aside.

2. To make salad, in a medium bowl add cooked, shredded chicken, diced celery, diced Granny Smith apple, finely chopped red onion and slivered almonds. Mix well. Pour dressing over the salad, toss to combine.

3. To assemble, fill a bowl with spinach leaves, cooked quinoa and curried chicken salad. Garnish with cilantro. Enjoy!

4. Store any extra curried chicken salad in an airtight container in the refrigerator for 3 to 4 days

Mashed Cauliflower with Rosemary Recipe.

Ingredients

* 1 large head of cauliflower

* 1 Tbsp. rosemary (chopped)

* 1.5 cups beef, chicken, or vegetable stock

* 3 garlic cloves (finely chopped)

* Salt and pepper to taste

Instructions

1. Place the stock and cauliflower in a medium saucepan and bring the boil, covered, for 15 minutes until the cauliflower is steamed and soft.

2. Place the cauliflower and stock in a blender, with the rosemary, garlic, salt, and pepper.

3. Blend on full power, stopping and scraping the sides, until smooth.

Braised Brussels Sprouts Recipe.

Ingredients

* 1 Tbsp. olive oil

* 3 shallots (sliced)

* 2 cloves garlic (crushed)

* 1 lb. Brussels sprouts

* 1 cup chicken or vegetable stock

* 4-5 sprigs fresh thyme (chopped)

* 1/4 cup pine nuts to top

* Salt and pepper to taste

Instructions

1. In a medium sized pan heat the oil over a medium heat.

2. Cook the shallots for 2-3 minutes until soft.

3. Add the garlic and cook for a further 2 minutes.

4. Add the sprouts and cook, stirring often, until brown patches appear on the sprouts.

5. Stir in the stock and thyme as well as salt and pepper to taste.

6. Cover and cook over a low heat for 10-15 minutes until sprouts are soft and tender, but not overcooked.

7. Top with pine nuts to serve.

Coconut Bread Stuffing Recipe.

Ingredients

* One loaf Candida Diet Coconut Bread, sliced and cut into 1 inch cubes

* 1 Tbsp. oil, coconut or olive

* 1/2 cup chopped celery

* 1/2 cup chopped onion

* 1/2 cup chopped mushrooms

* 1/2 cup thinly sliced leeks

* 1 tsp. dried thyme

* 1/2 tsp. salt

* Pepper to taste

* 1 cup water or vegetable/chicken broth

Instructions

1. Preheat oven to 325 degrees F (163 degrees C).

Brush an 8x8 casserole dish with oil, coconut or

olive, set aside.

2. Cut a loaf of Candida Diet Coconut Bread into 1 inch slices, then cut slices into 1 inch cubes. Place bread cubes into a large bowl, set aside.

3. Heat oil in a large skillet over medium heat. Add chopped celery, chopped onion, chopped mushrooms, and sliced leeks, saute for about 8 minutes.

4. Season vegetable mixture with dried thyme, salt and pepper, stir to combine. Add vegetable mixture and water or broth to bread cubes, gently stir to combine.

5. Place stuffing mixture in prepared casserole dish, cover and bake for 15 minutes. Uncover and

bake until stuffing is golden brown, about another

15 minutes. Serve warm.

Roast Turkey with Sage Pesto Recipe.

Ingredients

Sage Pesto

* 1 cup fresh sage leaves

* 1 tsp. finely minced garlic

* 1 tsp. lemon juice

* 1 tsp. lemon zest

* 2 Tbsp. hazelnuts

* 3 Tbsp. oil, olive or coconut, melted

* Salt and pepper to taste

Roast Turkey

* 1 bone in, skin on, half turkey breast (about 2

pounds)

* 1 Tbsp. oil, olive or coconut, melted

* 1/2 tsp. salt

* 1/4 tsp. pepper

Instructions

Sage Pesto

1. Add sage leaves, minced garlic, lemon juice and zest and hazelnuts to the bowl of a food processor. [SEP]

2. Process until mixture forms a paste, then add oil and process until mixture is smooth. [SEP]

3. Season pesto with salt and pepper to taste. Set mixture aside.

Roast Turkey

1. Preheat oven to 400 degrees (205 degrees C).

2. Place the half turkey breast in a large oven proof baking dish or on a rimmed baking sheet. With your fingers, carefully separate the skin from the turkey breast and spread sage pesto under the skin. Drizzle oil over the turkey breast, season with salt and pepper.

3. Roast the half turkey breast until a thermometer inserted into the center of the breast reaches 140 degrees (60 degrees C). That

should take about 30 minutes. [SEP]

4. Remove from pan, cover and let rest for 15 minutes. Slice turkey breast as needed, and drizzle with pan drippings if desired

Moroccan Stir Fry Recipe.

Ingredients

* 1/2 cup minced onion

* 1 clove garlic, thinly sliced

* 1 lb ground turkey

* 1 tsp. allspice

* 2 tsp. cumin

* 1 tsp. salt

* Pinch of pepper

* 2 cups roughly chopped chard leaves

* 2 cups thinly sliced green cabbage

* 2 Tbsp. minced fresh mint

* 1 orange bell pepper sliced into strips

* Zest of 1 lemon

* 1 Tbsp. lemon juice

* Plain yogurt for garnish

* Mint leaves for garnish

Instructions

1. In a large skillet over medium heat, add a bit of oil, olive or coconut, minced onion and sliced garlic. Sauté until the garlic is fragrant, about 1 to 2 minutes.

2. Add ground turkey, allspice, cumin, salt and

pepper to the skillet. Continue to sauté mixture until the turkey has browned, about 7 to 8 minutes.

3. Add roughly chopped chard leaves, thinly sliced green cabbage and orange bell pepper strips to meat mixture. Sauté until chard and cabbage have wilted and pepper strips have softened, about 3 minutes.

4. Add lemon juice and zest and give mixture a final stir.

5. Serve with a garnish of yogurt and fresh mint leaves

Celeriac Soup Recipe.

Ingredients

* 1 Tbsp. oil, olive or coconut

* 1 leek, white and light green parts, cleaned and

thinly sliced crosswise

* 1 celeriac, about 1 1/2 pounds, peeled and cut

into 1 inch dice

* 1/4 cup peeled, diced Granny Smith apple

(optional)

* 5 cups water

* 1/2 tsp. salt

* 1 tsp. dried thyme leaves

* Pepper to taste

* Fresh thyme leaves for garnish

Instructions

1. Heat oil in a large saucepan over medium heat.

Add leeks and cook, stirring, for about 5 minutes.

2. Add celeriac and apples (if using) and cook, stirring, for another 5 minutes.

3. Add water and bring to a simmer, then cover and cook until celeriac is tender, about 30 minutes.

4. Puree soup mixture until smooth in an upright blender, food processor or directly in the saucepan with an immersion blender.

5. Stir in dried thyme leaves, pepper to taste and additional salt if necessary.

6. Serve soup with a garnish of fresh thyme leaves.

Tarragon Chicken and Leeks Recipe.

Ingredients

* 1 4 oz. boneless, skinless chicken breast

* 1/2 teaspoon dried tarragon

* salt and pepper

* 2 Tbsp. oil, such as coconut or olive, divided

* 1 leek

* 1/2 cup water or chicken broth

* 1/4 cup canned unsweetened coconut milk

* Salt and pepper to taste

* Fresh tarragon for a garnish

Instructions

1. Place chicken breast between two sheets of plastic wrap or wax paper and pound with a meat mallet to about a 1/2 inch thickness. Season both sides of breast with dried tarragon, salt and

pepper, set aside.

2. In a large skillet over medium high heat, add a tablespoon of oil, such as olive or coconut. Sauté chicken breast until lightly browned on both sides and juices run clear, about 2 minutes per side. Transfer chicken breast to a plate, cover loosely with foil.

3. Trim away dark green leaves and root end of leek. Split leek in half lengthwise and rinse under running water, separating layers, to wash away any dirt.

4. In the same skillet over medium heat, add remaining tablespoon of oil. Place leek halves cut side down in skillet and sauté for 5 minutes. Add

water or chicken broth to skillet, cover and cook until leeks are tender and nicely caramelized, about 15 minutes. Transfer leeks to platter with chicken breast.

5. Add unsweetened coconut milk to skillet, scraping brown bits from bottom of pan with a wooden spoon. Simmer until sauce has heated through, about 2 minutes, then season with salt and pepper to taste. Pour sauce over chicken breast and leek halves. Garnish dish with fresh tarragon, serve immediately.

Tasty Salmon Bowl With Arugula Dressing Recipe.

Ingredients

Salmon Bowl

* 1 4-ounce salmon fillet

* 1/4 teaspoon dried sage

* Salt and pepper to taste

* 1 tablespoon oil, olive or coconut, melted

* 2 cups water

* 1/4 teaspoon salt

* 2 ounces fresh green beans, stem end trimmed

* 1/2 cup cooked tricolor quinoa

* 1 cup arugula, packed

* 2 ounces yellow pepper, thinly sliced lengthwise

* Blueberries (optional 'maybe' food)

* Pumpkin seeds

Arugula Dressing

* 2 cups arugula, packed

* 1 clove garlic, minced

* 1 1/2 tablespoons fresh lemon juice or apple

cider vinegar

* 1/4 cup olive oil

* Salt and pepper to taste

Instructions

Salmon Bowl

1. Heat oven to 400 degrees F (205 degrees C).

Place salmon fillet, skin side down, on a rimmed

baking sheet drizzled with oil. Season with dried sage, salt and pepper and roast until just cooked through, about 12 minutes. Remove salmon filet from oven, set aside.

2. In a small saucepan, bring water and salt to a boil. Add green beans and blanch just until bright green and tender crisp, about 2 minutes. Drain green beans and rinse under cold water for 1 to 2 minutes, set aside.

4. To assemble bowl, first add arugula and cooked tricolor quinoa, then top with roasted salmon filet. Next add green beans and sliced yellow pepper to the side, then drizzle with Arugula Dressing (see recipe below). Finally garnish bowl with a few blueberries (optional 'maybe' food) and pumpkin

seeds.

Arugula Dressing

1. In the bowl of a food processor, add arugula and minced garlic and pulse until finely chopped. Add lemon juice or apple cider vinegar and process until smooth. With the food processor running, drizzle in olive oil to make a smooth dressing. If necessary, thin with a bit of water to desired consistency.

2. Season with salt and pepper to taste. Refrigerate unused portion.

Asian Steak Kebabs Recipe.

Ingredients

Ingredients For Marinade

* 1/3 cup coconut aminos

* 2 Tbsp. water

* 1 Tbsp. sesame oil

* 6 drops liquid stevia

* 2 cloves garlic, minced

* 2 green onions, thinly sliced

* 1 Tbsp. sesame seeds, toasted

* 1 tsp. red pepper flakes

Main Ingredients

* 2 pounds steak, cut into 2 inch cubes

* 12 bamboo skewers (soaked in water for 30 minutes)

* Romain lettuce leaves

* Radicchio, cut in half, then thinly sliced

* Green onions, thinly sliced

* Sesame seeds, toasted

Instructions

1. Place all ingredients except steak cubes into a small bowl, whisk to combine, set aside.

2. Place steak cubes in an 8 x 8 glass baking dish, then add marinade and toss to coat. Cover baking dish with plastic wrap and marinate steak cubes for at least 2 hours or up to 24 hours in refrigerator.

3. Preheat grill, charcoal or gas, to medium-high heat. Thread steak cubes onto soaked bamboo skewers. Grill steak kebabs on a clean, oiled grate for about 3 to 4 minutes per side.

5. Transfer kebabs to a platter. Serve on lettuce leaves with thinly sliced radicchio and green onions and a sprinkle of sesame seeds. Coconut aminos with a sprinkle of red pepper flakes can be used as a dipping sauce.

Kimchi Meatballs Recipe.

Ingredients

Meatballs

* 1 Tbsp. olive oil

* 1 lb. ground turkey

* 2 scallions, finely minced

* 1 clove garlic, finely minced

* 1 Tbsp. fresh cilantro, finely minced

* 1 egg yolk, lightly beaten

* 1 tsp. sesame oil

* 1 tsp. ginger, freshly grated

* 1/2 tsp. salt

* 1/2 tsp. pepper

* 3 Tbsp. kimchi, minced

Sauce & Garnish

* 2 Tbsp. coconut aminos

* 2 Tbsp. sesame oil

* 0.5 cucumbers, cut into 24 slices

* 4 radishes, cut into 24 slices

* 1 Tbsp. sesame seeds

* 2 Tbsp. cilantro, finely minced

Instructions

1. Preheat oven to 400 degrees F (205 degrees C). Brush a rimmed baking sheet with a tablespoon of oil, set aside. [SEP]

2. In large bowl, mix together ground turkey, finely minced scallions, garlic and fresh cilantro, lightly beaten egg yolk, sesame oil, fresh grated

or powdered ginger, salt, pepper and minced kimchi. With wet hands, form meat mixture into 24 meatballs. Place meatballs on oiled baking sheet, about an inch apart and bake 20 minutes. Remove meatballs from oven, cool slightly.

3. In a small bowl, whisk together coconut aminos and sesame oil, set aside.

4. To assemble appetizer, place a radish slice on top of a cucumber slice, then top with a meatball, repeat to make 24 appetizers. Drizzle coconut amino/sesame oil mixture over the meatballs. Garnish appetizers with sesame seeds and finely minced cilantro

Buckwheat And Brussels Sprout Salad Recipe.

Ingredients

* 2 cups water

* 1 cup whole buckwheat groats

* Pinch of salt

* 2 Tbsp. oil, such as extra virgin olive or coconut

* ¼ cup shallots, thinly sliced

* ¼ cup celery, thinly sliced

* 1 clove garlic, minced

* 8 Brussels sprouts, cut in half lengthwise

* 1 Tbsp. fresh thyme leaves (or 1 teaspoon dried thyme)

* 1 cup vegetable broth or water

* Salt and pepper to taste

* 2 to 3 leaves Swiss chard, cut across into ribbons

* Fresh herbs, such as thyme or parsley, minced

* Crushed, toasted nuts, such as hazelnuts, pecans or walnuts

Instructions

1. In a medium saucepan, bring water and salt to a boil. Add whole buckwheat groats, cover and simmer for 15 to 20 minutes. Remove from heat, let rest for 5 minutes, fluff with a fork.

2. While buckwheat groats are simmering, heat oil in a large skillet over medium heat. Add shallots, celery, garlic, Brussels sprouts and saute until vegetables begin to soften and brown (about 5 minutes). Next, add fresh or dried thyme leaves, broth or water, salt and pepper to taste and simmer covered over medium low heat for about 10 minutes. Then add the Swiss chard, stirring to

wilt for about 1 to 2 minutes. Lastly, add cooked buckwheat groats to the skillet, and stir to combine.

3. To serve, you can garnish with fresh minced herbs and crushed, toasted nuts. For a salad, cool it to room temperature and toss with 2 to 3 tablespoons of extra virgin olive oil and 1 tablespoon of lemon juice.

Satay Chicken Bowl With Almond Sauce Recipe.

Ingredients

INGREDIENTS FOR CHICKEN SATAY BOWL

* 8 ounces boneless, skinless chicken breast or chicken tenders, partially frozen, cut into 1 inch cubes

* Zest and juice of 1 lime

* 1 Tbsp. coconut aminos

* 1 clove garlic, thinly sliced

* 1 tsp. ginger, fresh grated

* ¼ tsp. powdered turmeric

* 1 Tbsp. olive oil

* Salt to taste

* 1 cup cooked quinoa

* 2 cups mixed greens

* ½ cup thinly sliced red cabbage

* ¼ cup each of green onion, celery, cucumber, and yellow pepper, thinly sliced

* 2 Tbsp. slivered almonds

* Fresh cilantro and Thai basil, finely minced

* Lime wedges

INGREDIENTS FOR ALMOND SAUCE

* ¼ cup almond butter

* ¼ cup canned coconut milk

* 2 Tbsp. fresh lime juice

* 2 Tbsp. coconut aminos

* ¼ tsp. minced garlic

* ¼ tsp. powdered stevia

* 1 pinch red pepper flakes

Instructions

DIRECTIONS FOR CHICKEN SATAY BOWL

1. Cut partially frozen boneless, skinless chicken breast or chicken tenders into 1 inch cubes, set aside.

2. In a medium bowl, add lime zest and juice, coconut aminos, sliced garlic, grated ginger and powdered turmeric, whisk to combine. Add cubed chicken, toss to coat, cover and refrigerate 8 hours or overnight.

3. In a medium skillet, heat olive oil over medium high heat. Add chicken and cook until nicely browned on all sides, about 7 to 10 minutes. Remove chicken from skillet, season with salt to taste, set aside.

4. In a small bowl, add thinly sliced red cabbage, green onion, celery, cucumber, yellow pepper and slivered almonds. Toss to combine, set aside.

6. Divide all ingredients, cooked chicken cubes, quinoa, mixed greens, mixed vegetables/slivered almonds, between two bowls, arranging in sections as shown in photo. Garnish with finely minced cilantro,Thai basil and lime wedges. Serve immediately with Almond Sauce (see below) on the side.

DIRECTIONS FOR ALMOND SAUCE

1. Combine all ingredients in a small saucepan. Simmer sauce over medium heat, 2 to 3 minutes, whisking constantly until smooth and creamy, remove from heat.

2. If necessary, thin with 1 to 2 tablespoons of water or 1 tablespoon each of coconut aminos and fresh lime juice.

3. Serve sauce warm or at room temperature. Garnish with a pinch of red pepper flakes. If not using right away, store in an airtight container in the refrigerator.

Thai Quinoa Recipe.

Ingredients

* 1 cup quinoa, white, red, black or tricolor

* ½ cup unsweetened coconut milk

* ½ cup water

* Pinch of salt

* 2 Tbsp. coconut aminos

* 1 Tbsp. lime juice

* Juice from a 1 inch piece of ginger, peeled, finely grated, squeezed

* Salt to taste

* Red onion, thinly sliced

* Cilantro, finely minced

* Thai basil, finely minced

* Macadamia nuts, crushed

* Pink pepper corns, crushed

* Lime wedges

Instructions

1. Place quinoa, unsweetened coconut milk, water and salt in a medium saucepan and bring to a boil over high heat. Reduce heat to low, cover saucepan and cook quinoa for 15 minutes. Remove saucepan from heat, keeping quinoa covered for 5 additional minutes to absorb remaining liquid. Fluff quinoa gently with a fork, set aside to cool slightly.

2. In a small bowl whisk together coconut aminos, lime juice and ginger juice, season to taste with salt if needed.

3. In a large bowl add quinoa and coconut amino/juice mixture, toss to coat.

4. On a serving platter arrange in layers quinoa, red onion slices, minced cilantro and Thai basil, crushed macadamia nuts and pink peppercorns. Serve with lime wedges.

Yellow Squash Noodles with Meatballs and Olive Tapenade Recipe.

Ingredients

INGREDIENTS FOR YELLOW SQUASH NOODLES WITH MEATBALLS

* ½ lb. ground beef

* 2 Tbsp. onion, finely chopped

* 1 clove garlic, minced

* 1 Tbsp. fresh parsley, finely minced

* 1 egg yolk

* ½ tsp. salt

* ¼ tsp. pepper

* 4 Tbsp. oil, such as olive or coconut

* 2 medium yellow squash cut into noodles with a

spiral slicer, julienne peeler or mandolin

* 2 Tbsp. Olive Tapenade (see recipe below)

* Minced fresh parsley or basil for garnish

INGREDIENTS FOR OLIVE TAPENADE

* 1 cup black olives, packed in water

* 2 Tbsp. olive oil

* 2 tsp. lemon juice

* 1 clove garlic, minced

* Salt

Instructions

DIRECTIONS FOR YELLOW SQUASH NOODLES WITH MEATBALLS

1. Preheat the oven to 250 degrees F (120 degrees C).

2. In a large skillet, heat 1 tablespoon of oil over medium heat. Sauté onion for three minutes or until it becomes translucent. Then add garlic and

sauté for one minute. Remove skillet from heat, set aside.

3. In a large mixing bowl, add ground beef, sautéed onion and garlic, minced parsley, egg yolk, salt and pepper and mix until just combined. Divide meat mixture into 8 to 10 equal portions, depending on how large or small you want your meatballs. Roll each portion into balls.

4. Heat 2 tablespoons of oil over medium heat in the same skillet used to sauté onion and garlic. Brown meatballs on all sides, about 8 to 10 minutes. Transfer meatballs to a platter and keep in warm oven until ready to serve.

5. Wipe out skillet with paper toweling. Heat

remaining tablespoon of oil over medium heat. Add yellow squash noodles and cook for 2 to 3 minutes or until just tender. To finish, add 2 tablespoons of Olive Tapenade and a splash of olive oil, then toss to coat.

7. To serve, divide the yellow squash noodles onto two plates, top with meatballs, a spoonful of tapenade and a garnish of minced fresh parsley or basil.

DIRECTIONS FOR OLIVE TAPENADE

1. In the bowl of a food processor, combine all ingredients and pulse mixture until it resembles a

coarse paste.

2. Store tapenade in refrigerator in an airtight container for up to 2 weeks.

Sardine Nicoise Salad Recipe.

Ingredients

INGREDIENTS FOR NICOISE SALAD

* 2 cups water

* ¼ tsp. salt

* 2 ounces fresh greens beans, stem end trimmed

* 1 4-ounce can of boneless, skinless, sardines, drained

* 2 to 3 Romaine lettuce leaves, cut into bite size

pieces

* ½ tomato, quartered

* 1 hard boiled egg, quartered

* ¼ cup black olives, packed only in water and
salt

* ¼ cup cucumber slices, cut into half moons

* Fresh herbs such as oregano and chives, finely
minced

* Salt and pepper to taste

INGREDIENTS FOR THE ANCHOVY VINAIGRETTE

* 2 Tbsp. fresh lemon juice

* 6 Tbsp. extra virgin olive oil

* 2 anchovy fillets, finely minced

* Salt and pepper to taste

Instructions

1. In a small saucepan, bring water and salt to a boil and blanch green beans just until bright green and tender crisp, about 2 minutes. Drain green beans and rinse under cold water for 1 to 2 minutes.

2. Put the vinaigrette ingredients into a container with a lid, shake well. Refrigerate unused portion.

3. Arrange around a platter in separate mounds, the tomatoes, green beans, lettuce, hard boiled egg, cucumbers and olives. Place sardines in the middle of the platter and garnish with fresh herbs. Drizzle salad with the Anchovy Vinaigrette and season with salt and pepper to taste.

Oven Roasted Artichokes with Lemon and Olive Oil Dipping Sauce Recipe.

Ingredients

* 1 lemon, juiced

* 3 artichokes

* 6 tsp. and 3 Tbsp. olive oil, divided

* 2 cloves of garlic, thinly sliced

* Salt and pepper to taste

* Fresh herbs, such as thyme, oregano or parsley, finely minced

Instructions

1. Preheat oven to 400 degrees F (200 degrees C). Line a rimmed baking sheet with parchment paper, set aside. Place the juice of one lemon into a shallow dish, set aside.

2. Working with one artichoke at a time, begin by trimming one inch off the top of the artichoke. Cut a half inch off the stem end, then peel stem leaving only the tender inner stem. Remove any

lower, discolored leaves. Cut artichoke in half lengthwise and scoop out the choke, the fuzzy center, with a spoon. Dip cut side of artichoke halves in lemon juice to keep from browning. Repeat process with remaining artichoke halves. Save remaining lemon juice for dipping sauce.

3. Place artichoke halves on lined baking sheet, cut side up. Drizzle each half with a teaspoon of olive oil, sprinkle with salt and pepper. Place a few garlic slices in the center of each artichoke half, scatter over with fresh minced herbs. Turn halves over so the cut side is on the pan. Roast artichokes for 30 to 35 minutes.

4. While artichokes are roasting, make the dipping sauce by whisking together reserved lemon juice

and 3 tablespoons olive oil. Season with salt and pepper to taste.

5. Remove artichokes for oven, transfer to platter, serve with dipping sauce.

Cool Sardine Salad Recipe.

Ingredients

INGREDIENTS FOR SARDINE SALAD

* 1 4oz can boneless, skinless sardines, drained

* ½ cup thinly sliced fennel bulb

* ½ cup cucumber, peeled and small diced

* ¼ cup red onion, small diced

* ½ avocado, diced

* 2 Tbsp. Dill Vinaigrette (see recipe below)

* Salt and pepper to taste

* Chopped fresh dill for garnish

INGREDIENTS FOR DILL VINAIGRETTE

* 6 Tbsp. extra virgin olive oil

* 2 Tbsp. apple cider vinegar

* 1 Tbsp. fresh dill, finely minced

* Salt and pepper to taste

Instructions

DIRECTIONS FOR SARDINE SALAD

1. In a medium bowl add sardines and break them
up a bit with a fork.

2. Add sliced fennel bulb, diced cucumber, red onion and avocado and Dill Vinaigrette, toss.

4. Season with salt and pepper to taste, garnish with fresh dill and serve.

DIRECTIONS FOR DILL VINAIGRETTE

1. Put all ingredients into a container with a lid, shake well. Refrigerate unused portion.

Ajvar Dip Recipe.

Ingredients

* 1 eggplant

* 2 red bell peppers

* 1 clove finely minced garlic

* ¼ cup parsley, finely minced

* 2 Tbsps. lemon juice

* ¼ cup olive oil

* Salt and pepper to taste

Instructions

1. Heat oven to 475 degrees F (245 degrees C).

2. Place eggplant and peppers on a rimmed baking sheet and roast until skins begin to blacken, about 30 minutes. Place roasted vegetables in a plastic bag or in a covered bowl, let stand 10 to 15 minutes.

3. Peel skins off roasted vegetables, then place them into the bowl of a food processor along with the garlic, parsley, lemon juice and olive oil. Process all ingredients until mixture is smooth. Season with salt and pepper to taste.

4. Serve ajvar with a sprinkle of minced parsley. Store in a sealed container in refrigerator for up

to 1 week.

Buckwheat Ravioli Recipe.

Ingredients

MAKING THE FILLING

* 1 Tbsp. olive oil

* ½ cup finely chopped onion

* 1 clove finely minced garlic

* 1 pound ground meat, such as chicken or beef

* ½ pound greens, such as chard or spinach, stemmed and coarsely chopped

* ⅛ tsp. ground nutmeg

* Salt and pepper to taste

MAKING THE RAVIOLI

* 2 cups buckwheat flour

* ¼ tsp. salt

* 2 egg yolks

* 1 egg

* 1 Tbsp. olive oil

* Ravioli filling (see ingredients above)

Instructions

INSTRUCTIONS FOR THE FILLING

1. Heat olive oil in a large skillet over medium
heat.

2. Add the onion and garlic and cook until

softened, about 4 minutes.

3. Add the ground meat to the skillet and cook until browned, about 5 minutes.

4. Then add the greens and sauté until wilted, about 2 minutes.

6. Finally, add the ground nutmeg and salt and pepper to taste. Take skillet off heat, set aside.

INSTRUCTIONS FOR RAVIOLI

1. In a large bowl, add buckwheat flour and salt, whisk to combine. Make a well in the center of the flour mixture and add egg yolks, egg, olive oil and

water. With a fork, gently beat the egg mixture with out incorporating any of the flour mixture. Now with the fork, begin mixing in the flour mixture, a little at a time, with a stirring motion, until the dough is too stiff to mix with the fork.

2. Turn dough out onto a lightly floured surface, knead and shape dough into a smooth ball. If the dough is too dry, add more water, a tablespoon at a time, until dough is soft and pliable, but not too wet. Shape dough into a disk, wrap in plastic wrap and let it rest at room temperature for 30 minutes.

3. Working with half of the dough at a time, roll out to a 1/8 inch thickness, then cut into 3 inch circles. Spoon a tablespoon of filling onto the center of a dough circle, then moisten the edges

with water. Top with another dough circle and press along the edges until ravioli is firmly sealed. Set aside on a lightly floured surface. Repeat with remaining dough circles and filling.

4. Bring a large pot of salted water to a boil. Gently slide ravioli into the water and cook, a few at a time, until tender, about 5 to 7 minutes. Remove ravioli from pot with a skimmer, plate, serve with ajvar.

Nachos With Rutabaga Chips Recipe.

Ingredients

INGREDIENTS FOR RUTABAGA CHIPS

* 3 large rutabaga, peeled and sliced

* 3 Tbsp. oil, such as olive or coconut (melted)

* 1 tsp. salt

INGREDIENTS FOR SEASONED NACHO MEAT

* ½ Tbsp. oil, such as olive or coconut

* 1 pound ground meat, such as beef, bison or turkey

* 1 Tbsp. chili powder

* 2 tsps. onion powder

* 1 tsp. ground cumin

* 1 tsp. garlic powder

* 1 tsp. paprika

* 1 tsp. dried oregano

* 1 tsp. salt

* 1 cup water

INGREDIENTS FOR NACHOS

* Rutabaga chips

* Seasoned nacho meat

* Red pepper, seeded and diced

* Red onion, thinly sliced

* Green onion, thinly sliced

* Fresh cilantro, minced

* Guacamole

* Plain yogurt

Instructions

INSTRUCTIONS FOR RUTABAGA CHIPS

1. Preheat oven to 400 degrees F (205 degrees C).

2. Peel rutabagas, then with a sharp knife or mandoline, slice thinly. In a large mixing bowl, add rutabaga slices and oil, toss to coat evenly.

3. Spread slices in a single layer on a lightly oiled baking sheet, sprinkle with salt. Bake 25 to 30 minutes, flipping halfway to ensure even browning. Repeat with remaining rutabaga slices.

5. Transfer rutabaga chips to paper toweling to absorb excess oil. Chips will continue to crisp as they cool.

INSTRUCTIONS FOR SEASONED NACHO MEAT

1. In a large skillet, heat oil over medium heat.

2. Add ground meat and cook until browned, about 5 minutes, stirring occasionally to break up meat.

3. Add chili powder, onion powder, ground cumin, garlic powder, paprika, dried oregano and salt, stir to combine.

5. Add water, bring to a simmer and cook, uncovered, until liquid has evaporated, 15 to 20 minutes. Remove meat from heat.

FINISHING THE NACHOS

1. Place a layer of rutabaga chips on a plate. Spoon on seasoned meat mixture, top with guacamole and plain yogurt, then garnish with diced red pepper, sliced red and green onion and fresh minced cilantro.

www.ingramcontent.com/pod-product-compliance
Lightning Source LLC
Chambersburg PA
CBHW070757260726
48660CB00005B/1665